Why We Live Longer with Higher Cholesterol Levels

By

Lynne D M Noble

Independently published 2018

Contents

About the Author

Lynne Noble was born in 1953 in Huddersfield, West Yorkshire. From a very early age, Lynne showed an interest in nutrition and genetics avidly reading any books that she could get her hands on at the time.

Initially, Lynne studied orthopaedics but events led her to work with the elderly mentally infirm. Here, her interest in neurodegenerative disorders and pain syndromes developed.

Lynne undertook rigorous programmes of study, completing her Cert Ed., (FE) BSc (Hons) and Adv. Dip Education simultaneously before moving onto her M.Ed.

From there she took further demanding programmes in Human Nutrition, Pharmacology, Neuroscience, Genetics and Immunology. During this time, she was given many prestigious awards for her academic work. It was noted then that Lynne was not afraid of tackling difficult subjects.

She began her law degree but ill health prevented her from pursuing this. However, in this time, she moved from being a foster parent to adoptive parent.

She has been instrumental in setting up projects in the community for disadvantaged groups.

She is a member of the Guild of Health Writers.

Now retired, she lives in a picturesque village in West Yorkshire with her husband. She enjoys gardening, watching her husband bowling and researching.

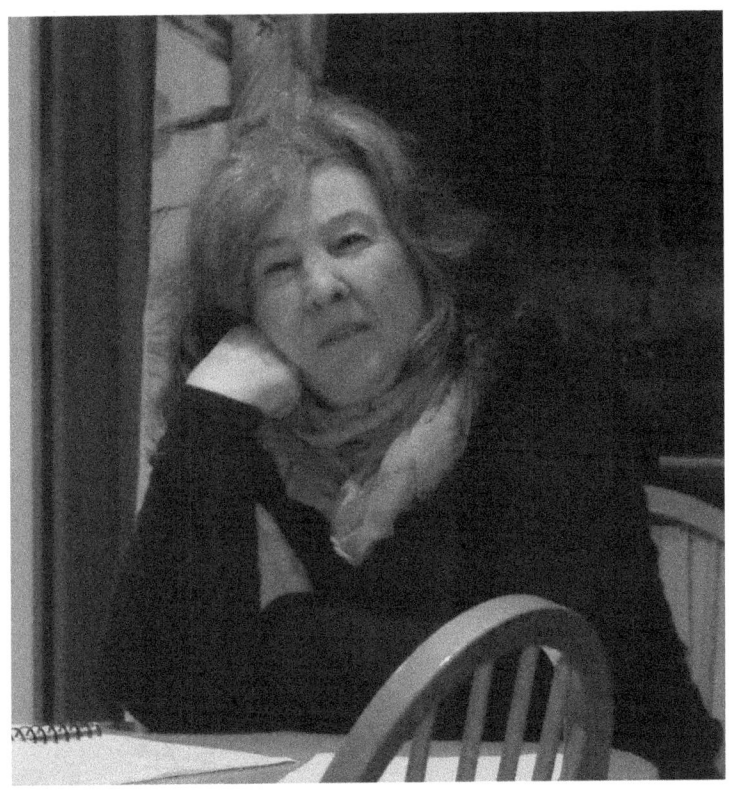

Author Lynne Noble at home

Forward

Many years ago I undertook a piece of research on memory decline. Research generally takes you into avenues that are not the main focus of your research but are intriguing enough to make you want to return to that particular area in the future.

My research led me to investigate cholesterol a little further. Sure, I had heard of it but didn't really know much about it, nor what it did. I had heard it was 'bad' and needed to be kept reined in by medication known as statins but, when I delved further, I came to understand just how much we need cholesterol in order to maintain a healthy and productive life. The impact on our health is so far reaching that this liquid gold and its demonization is incongruous with basic common sense.

My body of research grew and grew and, as it did so, I became more and more alarmed at the devastating damage on the human body that artificially lowering cholesterol levels, through taking statins, can do.

How did we come to an acceptance that mass medication of populations, with statins, has become the norm especially when all robust peer reviewed studies have demonstrated that high cholesterol levels are not responsible for cardiovascular events?

Indeed, we have been fed myths galore and they have become so much of our conversation that we now believe them with all our hearts. This is a dangerous thing to do. Look behind the hype and you will begin to see the falsehoods that have been perpetuated by those whose interests do not lie with the patients who will be fed statins.

Is there such a thing as good and bad cholesterol? Firstly, it has to be clarified that cholesterol is NOT LDL or HDL. Cholesterol is a waxy substance and, as it doesn't dissolve in blood it has to be carried on lipoproteins which transport it between cells. Lipoproteins are made up of an inner layer of fat and an outer layer of protein.

It is this 'raft' of LDL lipoprotein which is referred to as LDL or HDL and it is not cholesterol. The composition is entirely different. However, HDL and LDL have been used interchangeably so often with the word 'cholesterol' that the population now believes that they are one and the same.

Even low density lipoprotein – reputedly bad cholesterol - is associated with better cognitive functioning in older age provided it is the large fluffy LDL and not the small dense LDL. Perhaps you didn't know that there were different types of LDL and that some is so necessary for your health that to medicate it through the use of statins, is madness.

Tests do not distinguish between different types and, in fact, statins do reduce the good LDL – the sort that is required to help you form memories. Indeed, it is mentioned on the medication insert that some memory loss may occur through the use of your prescription.

The small dense LDL is able to slip through cells lining the wall of arteries and initiate inflammation and atherosclerotic changes but this is easily rectified through bespoke nutrition.

Therefore, statins are not required and, since they impact on other metabolic pathways, are not advisable as they can have life-changing consequences.

Total cholesterol is really a meaningless number unless it advises you of the different subtypes characterised by different particle sizes.

Most tests do not identify those so are useless as tests go.

Cholesterol has a diversity of amazing benefits for the human body but very few people will go out and seek this information for themselves.

For example, lowering cholesterol too much can lead to depression, negatively impact your sex life, cause muscle and nerve pain and increase your risk for cancer. Further, cholesterol secreted into the skin prevents it from cracking, keeps it smooth and wrinkle free. Cholesterol also transports fat soluble antioxidants around the body.

It is triglycerides that are the real culprit for cardiovascular disease. They are the storage form of fat and make the blood thick and sticky.

There is also a lipoprotein A that carries a sticky repair protein called apoliprotein. This is used for repair. It is a major risk factor for cardiovascular disease.

Why then, was cholesterol chosen to receive attention as a contributor to heart disease? Simply, it is a modifiable risk factor.

Before the 1920's cardiovascular disease was low in spite of a diet rich in butter, lard and dripping.

This book is intended to reveal the truth about cholesterol and statins. It will also reveal the real culprit behind cardiovascular disease and what an ordinary lay person can do to lower that risk. It will demonstrate why taking statins can shorten your life and be responsible for heart disease and how research has shown that taking statins can also dramatically increase your risk of neurodegenerative disorders.

This history of the encroachment of statins into a list of medicines which appear to be given out frequently is an interesting one. It is a history which is worth investigation if you have an enquiring mind. It is worth understanding the phrase 'modifiable risk factor.'

Basically, some medications are easier to produce than others to address certain issues. They may not necessarily be the best ones but simplicity often equals lower manufacturing costs and greater profits.

Out of a range of identified risk factors for any specific condition, the one that will be picked to address will most likely be the one that is cost effective.

This is true of most medications. You will note that if you go to the GP with an ailment, he will start you on a specific medication. If this does not work, they will work their way up a ladder of medications in a particular order. They will do this regardless of whether they feel that the last medication on the ladder, would be the best one to try as it is a better fit for the patient's symptoms.

Anyway, this book is intended to give you a little more knowledge about cholesterol, the medications required to treat it, dietary factors which can be used to lower any perceived rogue levels and whether medication is the right way to go for you.

As always, I advise taking a pen and paper and taking notes as you read this book so that you don't lose information which is of particular interest to you.

Firstly, we shall start off with a little history about the demonization of cholesterol.

The beginnings of the demonization of cholesterol

Some Facts

- 1953 Ancel Keys – biologist – proposed a radical theory that too much fat in the diet caused heart disease (Victorians who ate a very high fat diet had a very low incidence of heart disease but this passed him by).
- SEVEN COUNTRIES STUDY - Ancel Keys looked at the connection between fat consumption and heart disease of 22 countries. He selected seven countries which fitted his hypothesis and discarded the rest. This is known as statistical deception.[1]

---

[1] Statistical deception is used a lot to manipulate findings. For example, the absolute risk for someone with heart disease not taking statins is less than 1% but if you manipulate the statistics and produce them as the relative risk, this increases to between 30-50%

- When concerned researchers looked at the evidence from **all of** the countries in the study they found that there was no association between high fat diets or cholesterol with heart disease.
- John Yudkin – British researcher – found that the ONLY dietary factor that had the strongest link to heart disease was **sugar.**
- British Physician – Mendrick - found that if he chose another seven different countries that the more saturated fat and cholesterol consumed the lower the risk of heart disease.
- THE FRAMINGHAM HEART STUDY - conducted over 16 years of over 5,000 people in Massachusetts. This study showed that those who had heart disease and those who didn't had similar ranges of cholesterol. Lowering cholesterol levels for people who had heart disease only had any impact up to the age of forty- seven years. After the age of 48 years those with high cholesterol levels lived longer than

those with low cholesterol levels[2]. Further, the more saturated fat, cholesterol and calories eaten, the lower the person's serum cholesterol was AND they were more physically active!

Most of the studies showing the positive impact of cholesterol on human health have not been given the prominence that they deserve but in spite of being found wanting, they have still continued to inform medicine.

I would like to say that the prescribing of medicines always exists in a culture wholly dedicated to the welfare of the patient but I would be telling a lie. Political and economic concerns, take advantage of situations. In 2004, it was noted that:

the National Education Program lowered the 'optimal' cholesterol levels. Eight out of nine people on the panel had financial ties to the pharmaceutical industry. [3]

---

[2] https://www.bmj.com/content/371/bmj.m4266/rr-0
[3] The Great Cholesterol Myth, J Bowden and Stephen Sinatra

It is necessary to delve a little further into what cholesterol really is and why it is so important for all round health. This book will help you do just that.

Cholesterol: what it is and what it does

Cholesterol is a waxy substance which our bodies make naturally. It is made in the liver and is made in far greater quantities than we ever take in through diet. If we were to eat a high cholesterol meal our liver would just make less to restore the status quo. Cholesterol is an essential molecule without which there would be no life; virtually every cell in the body is capable of synthesising it.

Cholesterol is a major structural molecule which other major structural molecules are made from; as such it is a component in:

- o Bile acids which help to emulsify fats before digestion
- o Helps to make vitamin D which has hundreds of roles to play in the human body including bone building

- synthesising an antimicrobial called cathelicidin and regulating the immune system thereby reducing the chances of an auto immune disease.
- Steroid hormones (including sex hormones) are all cholesterol based.
- It forms part of the myelin sheath that surrounds nerves and helps to carry messages.
- Other steroid hormones produced from cholesterol include cortisol. This hormone helps to regulate blood sugar levels and defending the body against infection. Aldosterone, another hormone produced from cholesterol, helps retain salt and water in the body.
- Low density lipoprotein (LDL) cholesterol is required for forming memories. The information leaflets that accompany statins state that one of the side effects of statins is memory loss.
- Studies have shown that cholesterol neutralises toxins produced by bacteria. This may be why it is found at the site of

arterial injuries. Of course some pathogens are able to cross the blood brain barrier, invade the brain, instigate neuro-inflammation and consequently neurodegeneration. Other pathogens which normally do not cross the blood brain barrier may if the brain is injured in some way. This is what we are wanting to avoid in the first place. Cholesterol helps protect and repair the brain.

We shall look at some of the above in more detail later. Meanwhile it is probably better to dispel the myth of 'good' and 'bad' cholesterol. The LDL and HDL that most people are familiar with are actually lipoproteins – not cholesterol. That is, they are made from a combination of a fatty molecule (not cholesterol) and a protein molecule. Lipoproteins are like rafts carrying cholesterol to where it is needed (low density lipoprotein) or taking away any excess (high density lipoprotein raft) to the liver when it is not needed.

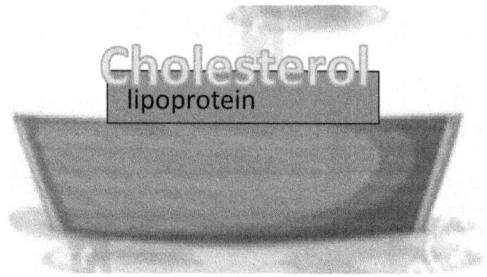

lipoprotein

Medics do not like LDL scores to be higher than HDL scores. However, there are numerous studies showing that high LDL is correlated with better memory and increased longevity.

A recent study found that better memory and thinking was found in the over 85's in spite of high cholesterol.[4]

---

[4] https://www.alzheimersresearchuk.org/better-memory-thinking-seen-85s-despite-high-cholesterol/

This has been replicated in other studies numerous times over.

In fact, it is the cholesterol carried on LDL – not HDL - that is linked with better cognitive function as you age. Why, in that case would you want to lower your LDL?

The best marker for the small dense LDL that is associated with atherosclerotic plaque is the C-reactive protein test or CRP test. This common test identifies inflammation which is associated with atherosclerotic plaque.

 The test that is given to determine cholesterol scores is entirely different. It is a simple test which looks at the levels of high density lipoprotein (HDL) and low density lipoprotein (LDL) in the blood. It assumes that all LDL contributes to disease, when this is far from the truth.

They don't distinguish between the beneficial and harmful types of LDL.

———————————————

C-reactive protein is a marker for inflammation. It is a strong indicator of future cardiovascular and neurological events.

High C-reactive protein can also be found during

- During times of high blood sugar levels
- Infection
- Obesity
- When blood is sticky (generally associated with high homocysteine (Hcy) levels.

I shall look at homocysteine, a little later among other substances that stimulate inflammation.

Did the well-respected Framingham Mass study reveal any alarming findings about cholesterol or saturated fat then?

William Castelli M.D. wrote this which appeared in the Archives of Internal medicine.

In Framingham Mass, the more saturated fat one ate, the more cholesterol one ate, the more calories one ate, the lower the person's serum cholesterol .... we found that people who ate the most cholesterol, ate the most saturated fat [and] ate the most calories, weighed the least and were the most physically active.

In spite of a robust trail of research that showed that cholesterol was vital for human health and optimal levels had been artificially lowered, manufactures jumped on the bandwagon and started producing plant based health drinks and margarines that promised to lower cholesterol levels. These, of course, came at a price.

The soluble fibre found in oatmeal, many fruits and lentils, for example, is applauded as being able to reduce levels of cholesterol. It can do this because it is not absorbed in the intestine and so binds to cholesterol and removes it from the body. Once manufacturers realised that their products could reduce cholesterol, the prices of their goods went up.

Of course, we had to be convinced first that LDL cholesterol was unhealthy and had to be dispensed with.

Lowering cholesterol levels, through the use of statins, has not been proven to have prevented even one heart attack. High cholesterol levels are associated with increased longevity and impact positively on the structure and function of the brain. Cholesterol, for example, has a critical role to play in the transmission of neurotransmitters.

This means that they pass messages on. Acetylcholine, for example, is necessary for motor control, learning, memory, sleep and dreaming. Low levels of acetylcholine have been found in those diagnosed with Alzheimer's disease.

Statins have been associated with an increase in motor neuron disease. Indeed, the sharp rise in ALS, the most common form of motor neuron disease which occurred in the 1990's, also coincided with the time when statins were heavily marketed.

Cholesterol is a vital component of the brain. Given the increasing numbers of neurodegenerative diseases in society at the moment, this subject deserves a chapter in itself.

Cholesterol is a vital component of the brain

As we have already ascertained, cholesterol has a bad press - like full fat milk, butter and egg yolks they've all been unfairly demonised. Anyone with a suggestion of a 'high' serum cholesterol level is generally offered statins in an effort to artificially lower their levels. Many others – and I know quite a few of these individuals – are given statins when their cholesterol levels, C-reactive protein levels and blood pressure levels are within current acceptable levels[5]. Statins are given as a 'preventative' measure. The body, at that point, appears to be healthy without any need for the alleged health benefits of taking statins.

If statins are taken when there is no need for them, the effect will be to reduce cholesterol

---

[5] Cholesterol levels were based on what was common' for Americans. The concentration results are plotted on histograms and the type of distribution established. The reference ranges are derived from the central 95th percentile.

levels below that which is required for maintenance and repair of the body.

Cholesterol has numerous functions in the body and is a **vital ingredient** for brain structure. By not supplying enough cholesterol, one of the potential outcomes is neurodegeneration and an inability to repair any injury to neural tissue.

I have spoken to many people who have had a blood test to check their cholesterol levels and who have subsequently been informed that their cholesterol levels are too high. They have been advised to take statins. Some have refused to do so and unfortunately a fairly high percentage of these individuals have been informed that if they refuse to take prescribed statins then they will need to find another GP.

Others have been offered one further blood test to ascertain whether their cholesterol levels are still high. This suggests to me that clinicians are aware of the fluctuating nature of cholesterol.

When the offer of a further blood test has been taken up, it has been found that the cholesterol score has lowered itself naturally without any medical intervention or the need for statins. How or why has this happened?

Serum levels of many substances, including cholesterol will vary depending on what has been recently eaten. A high cholesterol meal which might include prawns, for example, will increase serum cholesterol levels temporarily. If a blood test is taken shortly after the prawns have been eaten, then serum levels may appear abnormally high. A healthy functioning liver, however, is very efficient at bringing levels down to the body's requirements at the time, so it is only a temporary and easily adjustable event. However, within this lies another tale.

You could argue that the blood test is a fasting blood test and therefore the effects of the last meal really don't apply. However, fasting can be stressful......

Studies have also shown that stress contributes to a rise in cholesterol levels but quickly drops back once the stressful event is over. There is no great mystery about this – cholesterol is used in the formation of hormones including adrenaline. Adrenaline is needed to assist the body in coping with stress.

Adrenaline is made in the adrenal medulla of the adrenal glands and also in some neurons. Cholesterol has to travel to these target organs from the liver where it is made. Its transport system is the circulatory system so at times of stress when more adrenalin is required, then there will be a corresponding increase in serum cholesterol. This is not an abnormal response. It is an adaptive response.

At any point in time the body's demands for cholesterol may rise. It may be that an extra fat laden meal is eaten in which case extra bile is required.

To accommodate this short term event, serum cholesterol will rise as the body responds to the challenge of producing more bile. In fact, serum cholesterol levels may differ markedly throughout the day. The rhythmic rise and fall of serum cholesterol should not be a cause for concern.

My research that I undertook some time ago, showed the dangers of lowering cholesterol by taking statins. This piece of research – a literature review – showed:

- Higher levels of cholesterol are correlated with longevity.
- Low serum cholesterol is correlated with higher mortality.
- A 1mg fall of cholesterol in every dl of serum increased mortality by approximately 14% annually
- Those people with higher low density lipoprotein (supposedly the bad cholesterol) had better memories than those with low levels. In fact, there are higher rates of poor cognitive processing in those individuals with lower levels of cholesterol.
- In spite of popular belief, cholesterol has never been clinically proven to be the causative factor of any heart attack and

further, more than three quarters of individuals who have a heart attack have normal levels of cholesterol.

- Low levels of cholesterol are a clinically proven risk factor for a number of different types of cancer as well as respiratory and gastro intestinal diseases.
- Cholesterol supports the immune system by improving signalling in a set of cells known as Tregs. This helps fight inflammation. Studies have shown that increasing Tregs slows down the progression of motor neurone disease and other neurodegenerative disorders.
- Coffee intake has also been found to slow down the progression of MND. It is interesting to note that the intake of coffee is correlated with an increase in cholesterol levels – of about 10%. However, coffee also contains many potent antioxidants, too that could also account for this effect.

- Cholesterol helps absorb fat soluble vitamins ADEK
- It helps take up serotonin in the brain. Serotonin is a neurotransmitter which aids sleep
- Foods containing cholesterol are the main dietary sources of choline. This B vitamin is essential for the health of the liver, brain and nervous system.
- The greater the reduction in cholesterol levels, the greater the likelihood of a neurodegenerative disorder linked to a vitamin D deficiency. Cholesterol is required to synthesise vitamin D from the sun's rays. Vitamin D receptors are found throughout the brain and help to regulate any inflammatory processes.

It is clear that if cholesterol levels are artificially lowered through the use of medication that one or more of the areas, which require cholesterol for optimum health, are going to suffer.

Research continues to demonstrate that those with higher cholesterol levels have greater longevity, better memories and overall health, including more structurally healthy brains and nervous tissue. The cell body wall is made from cholesterol without which cells would collapse and die.

What is perhaps most chilling, is that researchers at the University of California and Advera Health Analytics inc. worked together to analyse data from the FDA Adverse Event Reporting System (FAERS) to determine what is known as reporting odds ratios (RORS) involving statin drug users who have reported ALS symptoms.

An ROR of two means the risk is twice as high.

The determination of likelihood of statin user's increased risk for ALS by statin products as found to be thus:

Table showing RORS for developing ALS type symptoms for specific statins.

Statin Drug Name –	ROR
Rosuvastatin	9.09 (809%)
Pravastatin	16.2 (1,502%)
Atorvastatin	17.0 (1,600%) *
Simvastatin	23.0 (2,200%) *
Lovastatin	107 (10,600%)

Most statisticians consider an ROR above six as a likely cause for a medical condition.

These findings[6] have been replicated by the World Health Organisation Foundation Collaborating Centre for International Drug Monitoring. They receive safety reports associated with statin medications and they have noted a disproportionately high number of patients with upper motor neuron lesions among those taking statin medications.

Statins work by inhibiting the enzyme your liver uses to produce cholesterol. However, the same pathway may also suppress the precursor to coenzyme Q10. This is an antioxidant that your mitochondria use to produce energy. When mitochondrial energy production is

---

[6]   https://link.springer.com/article/10.2165%2F00002018-200730060-00005

compromised. It may trigger - or accelerate - neuropathies like ALS.

In addition, Co enzyme Q10 is necessary for the production of collagen and elastin. It is a strong antioxidant and reduces the risk of blood clots and the rupture of fatty plaques in arteries.

A lack of Q10 results in muscle wasting and heart failure, neuropathy and inflammation of the tendons and ligaments.

Statins also dysregulate the Kappa Beta pathway. When the Kappa Beta pathway is compromised, there is a significantly increased risk of neurodegenerative disorders such as Alzheimer's Disease.

Statins impact on:

The Mevalonate pathway	involved in cholesterol production and sex hormones and adrenal hormones
The Kappa Beta Pathway	When it is dysregulated as happens with statin use then neuropathologies such as Alzheimer's occurs.
The Production of Co-enzyme Q10	When this is dysregulated through the use of statins then diseases like Alzheimer's occur

Isn't cholesterol a risk factor for heart disease?

The difference between risk factor and causation needs to be understood. Cholesterol has been identified as a risk factor for cardiovascular events in elderly men. Why would that be?

A risk factor is not causation.

At sites of injury, cholesterol is required for repair. It is the LDL that transports healing cholesterol to cells. Higher levels of LDL to HDL can alert us to the fact that there is an inflammatory process going on in the body. It is not causation.

So that they can repair themselves. What is required, when LDL levels are raised, is recognition that we need a test for levels of C-reactive protein to ascertain whether raised inflammatory levels are a cause for concern.

It also helps to establish the type of LDL through a test which shows the precise nature of LDL; that is, is it big and fluffy or small and dense.

Sometimes, an injury may have occurred that requires cholesterol for its repair and healing. Remember that cholesterol is an integral part of the cell membrane. Therefore, it is also needed for the repair and maintenance of cells.

Cholesterol is not the problem it is the **oxidisation**[7] of cholesterol and inflammation that can cause problems. However, it is not just cholesterol that oxidisation affects so it is strange that it has been singled out.

Oxidisation occurs everywhere in the body and a suitable response needs to be actioned if inflammatory levels are found to be unreasonably high.

For example, inflammatory processes that occur due to oxidisation require additional

_____

[7] Oxidisation – the addition of oxygen to a compound with a loss of electrons during this process.

antioxidants to be added in the diet to help with neutralisation of unpaired electrons.

Antioxidants are generally associated with diets high in fruit and vegetables. There are indeed many antioxidants in fresh fruit and vegetables. However, they also exist in foods sourced from animals.

Zinc is one such antioxidant. There is hardly any in foods of plant origins and what there is binds to phytates in plants and is not available for the body to use.

When you consider that zinc is used in the synthesis of over 300 enzymes and 800 macromolecules which are vital for the health of our body then we may begin to appreciate its impact.

At the moment there appears to be a leaning towards vegetarian and vegan diets and a cultural aversion to eating meat for many reasons.

However, we need to take a step back and look at this again.

Excessive oxidative stress is not only the cause of disease but the effect of a diverse range of pathological conditions such as diabetes, cardiovascular disease, cancers, neurodegeneration, to name just a few.

Increased oxidative stress is undoubtedly involved in ageing.

What is the food stuff that is related to oxidative stress? It is sugar. That stuff that Professor John Yudkin referred to in his book, 'Pure, White and Deadly' as being responsible for the increase in cardiovascular disease.

Selenium, a trace mineral, is another powerful antioxidant that is deficient in many diets due to selenium depleted soils that food is grown in.

The best sources are animal sourced food. Beans and peas will also contain some provided any soil deficiency of selenium has been addressed. Brazil nuts are by far the best source of selenium with one nut providing the daily allowance of this substance.

While it is easy to become deficient in selenium it is just as easy to suffer from toxicity if too many brazil nuts are eaten, for example. Not many nutrients have a such a narrow range that may cause problems if levels fall outside those parameters but selenium – and potassium – are two well-known ones.

What I hope that you take away from this, is that fruit and vegetables are not the only source of antioxidants although advertising leads heavily towards this.

In fact, fructose – the sugar found in fruit and vegetables can contribute to obesity and impair the optimum composition of blood lipids.

Numerous studies have demonstrated that fructose raises levels of Very Low Density Lipoprotein (another baddie) and this contributes to the accumulation of fat around the organs with a potential risk for heart disease.

Nevertheless, the Framingham Heart Study found that after the age of forty-seven, high levels of cholesterol were not a risk factor for cardiovascular disease.

In fact, studies have shown that low cholesterol levels are associated with heart arrhythmias. (heart rhythm irregularities).

Further, studies have found that statins themselves may stimulate atherosclerosis and heart failure through pharmacological mechanisms.

This potential for heart failure is not surprising. One of the well-known side effects of statins is their ability to break down muscle tissue. The heart is a muscle and just as susceptible to the effects of statins as any other muscle in the body.

Statins stimulate atherosclerosis and heart failure

One study presented a perspective that statins may be causative factor in coronary artery calcification as they function as mitochondrial toxins.

Firstly, statins   deplete Coenzyme Q10 and heme A followed by the depletion of a substance known as adenosine triphosphate (ATP) generation which helps to transfer energy within cells.

> Statins function as mitochondrial toxins and may promote arterial calcification

Coenzyme Q10 plays several vital roles in your body as well as synthesising and transferring energy within your cells. It is synthesised in every cell in the body.

Heme A gives myoglobin [8](muscle protein) and haemoglobin the ability to bind to oxygen because of the presence of the iron atom.

---

[8] https://www.ncbi.nlm.nih.gov/pubmed/25655639

Statins also inhibit the synthesis of vitamin K2 which protects arteries from calcification. Vitamin K2 also helps to regulate cholesterol levels.

Foods which contain vitamin K2 include butter, cheese and eggs. These are the very foods that we are told are bad for us.

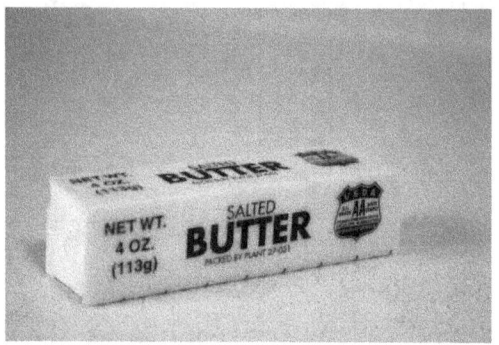

Statins inhibit the synthesis of vitamin K2 which protects arteries from calcification

Further, statins inhibit the biosynthesis of selenium containing proteins. An impairment of this may be a factor in the congestive heart failure that is associated with statin use. A selenium deficiency is known to result in dilated cardiomyopathy.

> Statins inhibit the biosynthesis of selenium containing proteins – this may be a factor in the congestive heart failure associated with statin intake.

The authors note:

The epidemic of heart failure and atherosclerosis that plagues the modern world may be paradoxically aggravated by the use of statin drugs.

The uptake of selenium, by plants, is poor due to selenium depleted soils. Nevertheless, as we have learned, two brazil nuts per day more than supply all your daily needs of selenium. As a timely reminder, it is not recommended that the recommended daily allowance is exceeded as selenium can be toxic in high does.

Other good sources of selenium are semolina, and mushrooms, as well as eggs and most meat sources.

Low cholesterol levels have not been found to increase survival rates in elderly men. Studies[9] have shown that low cholesterol levels increase the risk for growths, such as cancer, and other conditions not associated with cardiovascular events.

> Low cholesterol levels increase the risk for growths such as cancer

The increased risk for some cancers for statin users may be due to a number of reasons. This includes that our main form of vitamin D is synthesised from cholesterol by the action of the

---

9

https://www.ncbi.nlm.nih.gov/pubmed/12974874?ordinalpos=40&itool=EntrezSystem2.PEntrez.Pubmed.Pubmed_Results_Panel.Pubmed_DefaultReportPanel.Pubmed_RVDocSum

sun's rays on our skin.   A vitamin D deficiency results in a failure of the immune system to properly patrol for - and deal with - infections.

Many other studies[10] show that people with high cholesterol levels live the longest.

> Studies show that those people with high cholesterol levels live the longest

Studies[11] on women have found that the optimal cholesterol score is seven.   Mortality was found to be at its lowest at this level.

10

https://www.ncbi.nlm.nih.gov/pubmed/7246527?ordinalpos=8&itool=EntrezSystem2.PEntrez.Pubmed.Pubmed_ResultsPanel.Pubmed_DefaultReportPanel.Pubmed_RVDocSum

11

https://www.ncbi.nlm.nih.gov/pubmed/2564950?dopt=Abstract

In spite of this a cholesterol score of five or above is frowned upon by the medical profession. Patients are encouraged to take statins when a serum score of five is reached. The mass medication of the walking well has now begun.

There is also an increased risk of diabetes type 2 in those who are statin users.[12] Diabetes type 2 and cardiovascular disease are associated.

> There is an increased risk for Diabetes type 2 in those who are statin users.

In an online bulletin by Diabetes.co.uk in October 2017, it was reported that there was a 36% increased risk of diabetes type 2 among statin users.

---

[12] https://www.diabetes.co.uk/news/2017/oct/statin-use-linked-to-increased-risk-of-type-2-diabetes-94308054.html

This was a longitudinal study of 3234 individuals who had elevated BMI's and blood sugar levels. It is thought that statins impair insulin production.

Statins also reduce our ability to withstand infection. Studies[13] have found that statin users are more likely to contract methicillin resistant staphylococcus aureus (MRSA).

> Our ability to withstand infections is reduced with statin use

The authors of the study highlight that the epidermis is a very active site of cholesterol synthesis and after barrier disruption in a murine model, there was a brisk increase in cholesterol synthesis in epidermal cholesterol synthesis.

---

[13] https://www.mdedge.com/ccjm/article/94911/infectious-diseases/methicillin-resistant-staphylococcus-aureus-link-statin

They also noted that if the synthesis of cholesterol was inhibited by the application of statin as topical application, the barrier function was impaired.

Cholesterol is also required to neutralise bacterial toxins.

Bacterial toxins are virulence factors that target host cell function and hijack the processes so that microbial infection is able to flourish.

Some toxins directly target the innate immune cells and are able to wipe out the defensive action of the host immune response.

There is also an increased risk for post stroke infection in early statin use after such an event.[14]

Statins have also been found to significantly increase the risk of herpes zoster the reactivated virus. This the virus responsible for shingles.[15]

---

[14] https://www.ncbi.nlm.nih.gov/pmc/articles/PMC3202647/
[15] https://www.ncbi.nom.nih.gov/pmc/articles/PMO6001979/

Viruses are only reawakened when the immune system is below par. As there is an increased risk for respiratory and intestinal infections for statin users, then it appears that statins potentially have a negative effect on the immune system.

The American College of Cardiology reported a diversity of common statin side effects which are reproduced in the table below.[16] Surely, however, the potential impact of statins on health, should be a cause for alarm and raise questions about whether they should be prescribed at all.

---

[16] https://www.acc.org/latest-in-cardiology/articles/2015/08/11/09/16/statin-intolerance-not-a-myth

Table 1

Organ/Systems	Potential Side Effects of Statins
Respiratory	↑ risk of interstitial lung disease (0.01-0.4%), ↑ risk of upper respiratory tract infection (1-16%), ↑ risk of pharyngitis (3-13%), rhinitis (1-11%), sinusitis (2-7%), bronchitis (2%), cough (1-2%)
Neurologic and Psychological Effects	↑ risk of suicide, aggressive behaviour, ↑ headache (2-17%), asthenia (1-4%), dizziness (1-4%), fatigue (1-4%), ↑ risk of depressive disorder in stroke patients, ↑ risk of hemorrhagic stroke, severe irritability, insomnia, somnolence, agitation, confusion, hallucinations, and nightmares
Endocrine	↑ risk of new onset diabetes (NOD) (9-27%), Intensive-dose statin therapy is associated with a 12% higher incidence of NOD compared with moderate-dose statin therapy

Gastrointestinal Tract	↑ constipation, diarrhoea, dyspepsia, flatulence heartburn, nausea vomiting
Hepatic	< 1.5% hepatotoxicity in coronary artery disease patients in 5 years, ↑ liver enzyme activity
Skin	↑ risk of alopecia, lichenoid eruption, dermographism, chronic urticaria, toxic epidermal necrolysis and rash (1-4%)
Eye	↑ risk of cataract (up to 27%), ↑ diplopia, ptosis and ophthalmoplegia
Renal	↑ risk of acute renal failure, ↑ proteinuria
Reproductive	erectile dysfunction, decrease libido, gynecomastia , ⬇ testosterone levels (7.5-10.3%) after 48 weeks of statins
Blood	↑ risk of thrombotic thrombocytopenic purpura (TPP)
Bones and Joints	tendinitis, arthralgia, arthritis, lupus, polymyalgia rheumatica

Statins have become so much a part of our culture, that the mass medication of populations has become accepted as the norm.   This is regardless of whether patients have even had their cholesterol levels tested.

I am frankly horrified when I hear that patients have been prescribed statins as a preventative measure without any blood work to ascertain what their current levels are, anyway. I am equally horrified that patients' cholesterol scores are not regularly checked when they are on statins.

I would also ask what is trying to be prevented here?

Statins are associated with neurodegenerative disorders, increased risk of infection, heart disease, increased atherosclerosis, diabetes type 2, cognitive decline, a propensity to neurodegeneration, some cancers and increased mortality, among others.

 That doesn't sound much like preventing illness to me.

What could account for elevated levels of atherosclerosis?

In arterial plaque only 3% of it was found to be composed of cholesterol. However, calcium was found to contribute 50%[17] of the composition of arterial plaque.

A study published in Nature Immunology suggests that atherosclerosis is caused by macrophages. These are white blood cells that build up in arteries. Their job is to locate microscopic foreign bodies and eat them.

Nevertheless, due to the constant indoctrination of the alleged benefits of statins, the demonising of cholesterol and the failure of the populace to independently research their medication and consider the potential economic and political rationale for promoting these drugs, statins have become an accepted part of our lives.

Very few people will ever consider alternatives to statins if they do have an increased risk for heart disease. The main indicator – and cause of concern - for heart disease is increased blood pressure, not high cholesterol. High cholesterol

---

[17] S. Seely, 'Is Calcium Excess in Western Diet a Major Cause of Arterial Disease? (New York: Grand Central Life and Style, 2012)

scores indicate that there is a greater need of this substance in the body at that time. Increased serum cholesterol levels may be responding to the demands than an infection brings with it or it may be responding to low grade subclinical inflammation that occurs when blood sugar levels spike, for example.

If high blood pressure is in evidence, then there are a number of ways of addressing the increased risk for cardiovascular disease through sound nutrition and some simple lifestyle changes. None of these involve eating lettuce leaves or charging around the countryside on a wet summer's day in order to increase exercise.

Both of those suggestions are likely to raise most people's blood pressure!

It seems at this point a logical place to change focus and look at ways of decreasing risk for cardiovascular events and stroke without medication that lowers cholesterol levels.

The benefits of good nutrition

The benefits of good nutrition cannot be stated enough. The diversity of foods that are within our grasp will contain all the medicine that we need. In addition, we need sunshine and fresh air, moderate exercise, the time to relax - and follow our own pursuits - and to be surrounded by supportive and significant others, for optimal wellbeing.

When most people think of statins and cholesterol, it is in the context of 'what can this do for any cardiovascular risk I may have?' That is a good question to ask. Some people do not appear to have any risk for cardiovascular disease and yet are still pressed to take statins.

I met a lady on holiday recently. I shall call her Sue for this particular illustrative purpose. She was travelling with her 90-year-old mother who was very fit and healthy and who had older siblings who were also fit and healthy. All of them had raised cholesterol levels (by today's standards) and yet none had had any cardiovascular event or stroke. There was no hint of any cognitive decline in our ninety-year-old and we enjoyed many a stimulating conversation.

Sue – who was a very young looking 60-year-old - had been informed that her cholesterol levels were raised. They were in line with her mother's - and aunts - scores.

Sue had been pressed by her GP to go on statins and Sue did not want this. She had changed her diet and become vegetarian promising the GP that she would be 'good.' She pleaded with me to help her lower her cholesterol levels while acknowledging that her mother and aunts were very fit and healthy with their high cholesterol scores.

In the end Sue reluctantly went on statins. She knows that this is not wise but the pressure of cultural expectations - and the pressure from her GP - was just too much for her to cope with.

This story probably illustrates how much we now cannot shake off the belief that statins are good and cholesterol is bad, in spite of robust evidence to the contrary.

Vitamin K2

We have briefly looked at vitamin K2 as a potent 'medicine' for keeping arteries clean and lowering blood pressure. Most people have never heard of vitamin K2 never mind have an understanding of what this powerful vitamin can do to keep people heart healthy.

Vitamin K2 activates proteins that have a role in blood clotting and calcium metabolism, among others. Calcium deposition in arteries narrows arteries that subsequently will push up blood pressure. Studies have shown that vitamin K2 can reduce blood vessel calcification - thereby increasing the diameter of blood vessels - and lowering blood pressure in the process.

A long term study[18] has shown that people with the highest intake of vitamin K2 were 52% less likely to develop artery calcification and had a 57% lower risk of dying from heart disease.

Another study[19] that involved nearly 17,000 women found that participants with the highest intake of vitamin K2 had a decreased risk of heart disease. It was found that for every 10mcg of K2 that was consumed daily, the heart disease risk was reduced by 9%.

As well as preventing calcification, vitamin K2 also helps to prevent inflammation. Where injury due to inflammation occurs, the need for cholesterol increases. Cholesterol will be required for repair.

A Rotterdam study found that for men who followed a high K2 diet, this was associated with lower risks of severe aortic calcification, cardiovascular disease and cardiovascular mortality.

---

14 https://www.ncbi.nlm.nih.gov/pubmed/15514282
[19] https://www.ncbi.nlm.nih.gov/pubmed/19179058

This wonder vitamin is easily obtainable in diet, over the counter and online and does not carry with it the risks associated with statin use. It would be far preferable to increase the daily intake of vitamin K2 rather than accept a prescription for statins.

There are a number of conditions which predispose to a vitamin K deficiency and these are:

- Those who have coeliac disease
- Those who have cystic fibrosis
- Those who have had parts of their intestine remove
- Those who have diseases like Crohn's disease or problems with their liver, gall bladder and bile ducts
- Those people who have very low fat diets (unfortunately, low fat and no fat diets appear to be popular at the moment.

What foods contain this wonder vitamin?

Vitamin K2 can be found in:

- All fermented foods especially natto
- Cheese
- Eggs
- Butter
- Dark chicken meat
- Goose liver

In fact, most of the foods that are frowned upon if you want to avoid heart disease. It does illustrate how far we have lost sight of what is really healthy eating.

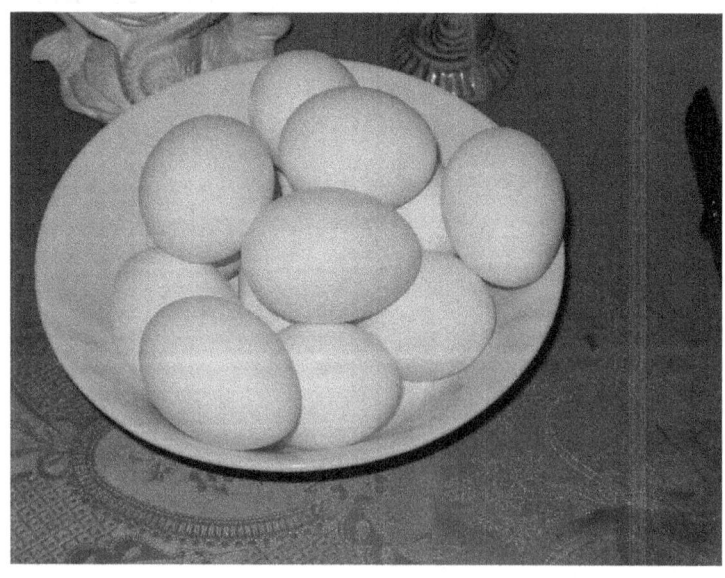

Eggs are full of heart healthy vitamin k2.

The recommended dietary allowance for women is 122mcg daily and 138 mcg for men.

As vitamin K is a fat soluble vitamin, it needs to be taken with a little fat for it to be absorbed in the intestine.

Magnesium

Magnesium is involved in many, many enzymatic actions in the body many of which are related to cardiovascular health. It has anti-inflammatory benefits and can prevent the build-up of inflammatory cells in arteries.

Magnesium is also able to dilate arteries which means there is less resistance to the blood as it flows through arteries. This lowers blood pressure.

Most people appear to have some degree of magnesium deficiency nowadays. The original recommended dietary allowance daily was 400mg but this has recently been increased.

Good sources of magnesium are:

- Dark chocolate
- Nuts
- Seeds
- Whole grains
- Dark green leafy vegetables such as spinach, chard, kale

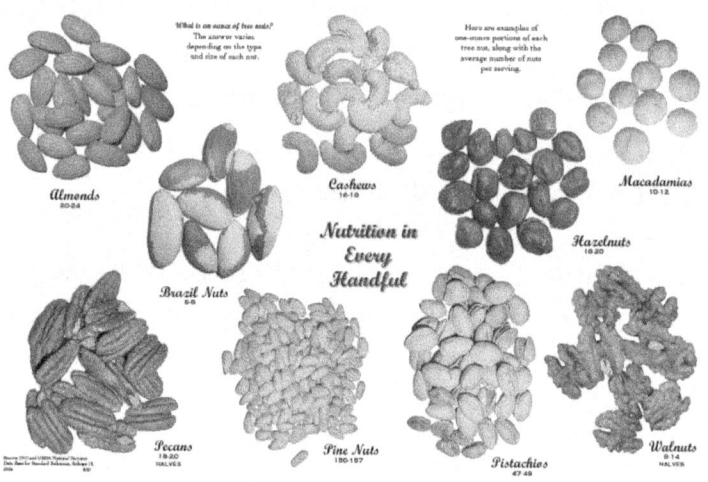

Copper

When I ask people what they think copper's function is in the body, they generally have no idea. However, copper is a necessary trace mineral for heart health.

Some studies have suggested that some patients with heart failure may benefit from copper supplements. Further, animal studies have linked low copper levels with cardiovascular disease but whether these results can be extrapolated to humans is unclear.

A 2018 study[20] argued that copper deficiency may be a leading cause of ischaemic heart disease. Ischaemic heart disease is where heart problems are caused by narrowed arteries. Narrowed arteries impede the flow of oxygen and nutrients that are vital for tissues to remain healthy.

---

[20] https://openheart.bmj.com/content/5/2/e000784

High intakes of copper will deplete zinc so a balance must be maintained. A deficiency of zinc is implicated in viral conditions like shingles.

The recommended dietary allowance for copper is 900mcg daily. Greater intakes of copper are not recommended. An excess as well as a deficiency can have harmful effects on the body.

Good sources of copper are:

- Liver and other organ meats
- Dark chocolate
- Dark leafy greens
- Cocoa
- Beans

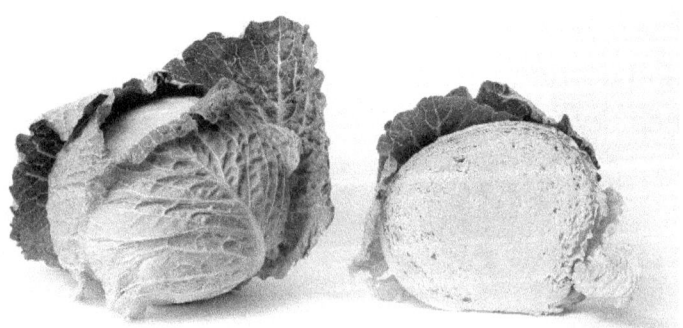

Selenium

A deficiency of selenium is detrimental to heart health as a deficiency has been linked to an increased risk of coronary heart disease. In an analysis of 25 observational studies[21], a 50% increase in blood selenium levels was associated with a 24% reduction in coronary heart disease.

The recommended daily amount for various age groups is seen in the table below

Group	Recommended Dietary Allowance
Children 1-3	20 micrograms/day
Children 4-8	30 micrograms/day
Children 9-13	40 micrograms/day
Adults and children 14 and up	55 micrograms/day
Pregnant women	60 micrograms/day
Breastfeeding women	70 micrograms/day

[21] https://www.ncbi.nlm.nih.gov/pubmed/17023702

Selenium is toxic in large amounts so this should be borne in mind. However, it is easy to become selenium deficient since most soils are. Therefore, plant content is poor.

Good sources of selenium are:

- brazil nuts (no more than two daily)
- semolina
- Yellow fin tuna
- All meats

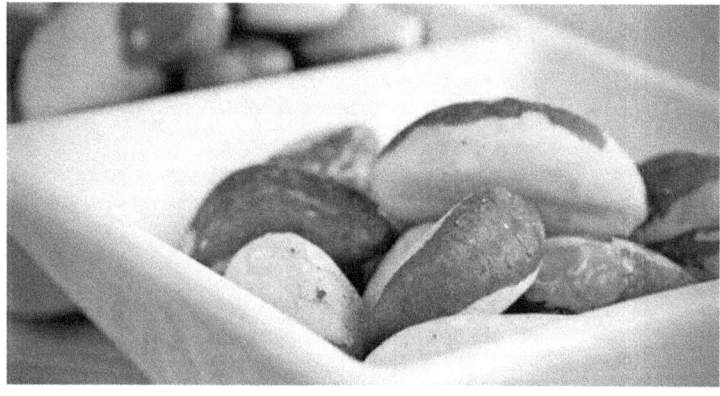

Brazil nuts contain excellent amounts of selenium but no more than two a day are allowed.

Vitamin B complex and the methionine cycle

Methionine is an amino acid which is the substrate of many other substances such as cysteine and taurine which are also amino acids.

As it goes through its cycle, it briefly forms homocysteine. Homocysteine is an amino acid that can have damaging and inflammatory effects on tissues of the body including arteries. Fortunately, its conversion back to methionine happens fairly rapidly provided three important B complexes are available. These are vitamins B6 and B9 and B12. Vitamin B9 is more commonly known as folic acid.

However, if the above vitamins are not available then homocysteine will certainly damage the delicate artery linings. They will be 'roughened up' in the process.

Further, excessive homocysteine causes 'sticky blood' and reduces the flexibility of blood vessels. When damage occurs the inflammatory process attracts substances required for repair of the injury.

The   inflammation that ensues narrows blood vessels. Narrowed arteries increase blood pressure. The heart is forced to work harder than it should.

There is a direct correlation between high homocysteine levels and an increased risk of heart disease and stroke.

One study looked at over 3000 patients with elevated levels of homocysteine. It was found that a subsequent coronary event was 2.5 times more likely in those with elevated levels of homocysteine.

It was also found that for each increase of 5 micromoles per litre of homocysteine there was a predicted 25% increased risk of coronary events.

Further, there is always the potential - for any of the substances involved in the repair - to break off and travel to much smaller arteries. If the oxygen supply is cut off in the process, then a cardiovascular event will result.

Folic acid (400mcg per day), vitamin B6 (25 to 100mg per day) and vitamin B12 (2-100mcg) per day have been shown to break down homocysteine that is linked to an increased risk of heart disease and stroke. This high dose vitamin supplementation has been found to significantly reduce the progression of early stage subclinical atherosclerosis.

However, it would be judicious to take the vitamin B complex in its entirety since they work synergistically   and vitamin B6, 9 and 12 by no means comprise the whole of the B complex.

While supplementation can be useful, I always recommend getting your nutritional needs from food sources, where possible.

Good sources of vitamin B complex are:

- Seeds
- Nuts
- Whole grains
- Brewer's yeast
- Red meat
- Brown rice

- Dark chocolate
- Dark green leafy vegetables

Vitamin B complex is water soluble and easily leaches away in the cooking processes. It is also easily destroyed with heat.

Vitamin B12 needs an acidic environment to be removed from its source. Consequently, those on antacids may find that they are deficient in vitamin B12.

As already stated, vitamin B complex is water soluble and easily flushed away in urine.

Drugs which may raise levels of homocysteine

There are a number of prescribed medications that have a tendency to elevate homocysteine levels. These are:

- Theophylline – prescribed for asthma
- Methotrexate – for cancer or arthritis
- L-Dopa – for Parkinson's disease

If you are prescribed any of these drugs, then it is judicious to have homocysteine levels tested on a regular basis and include more of the vitamin B complex in your diet.

Supplemental vitamin B is easily available in supermarkets and does not cost a great deal. You do not need to buy expensive brands.

Brewer's yeast is also a good source of the B complex but has the added benefit of containing selenium, too.

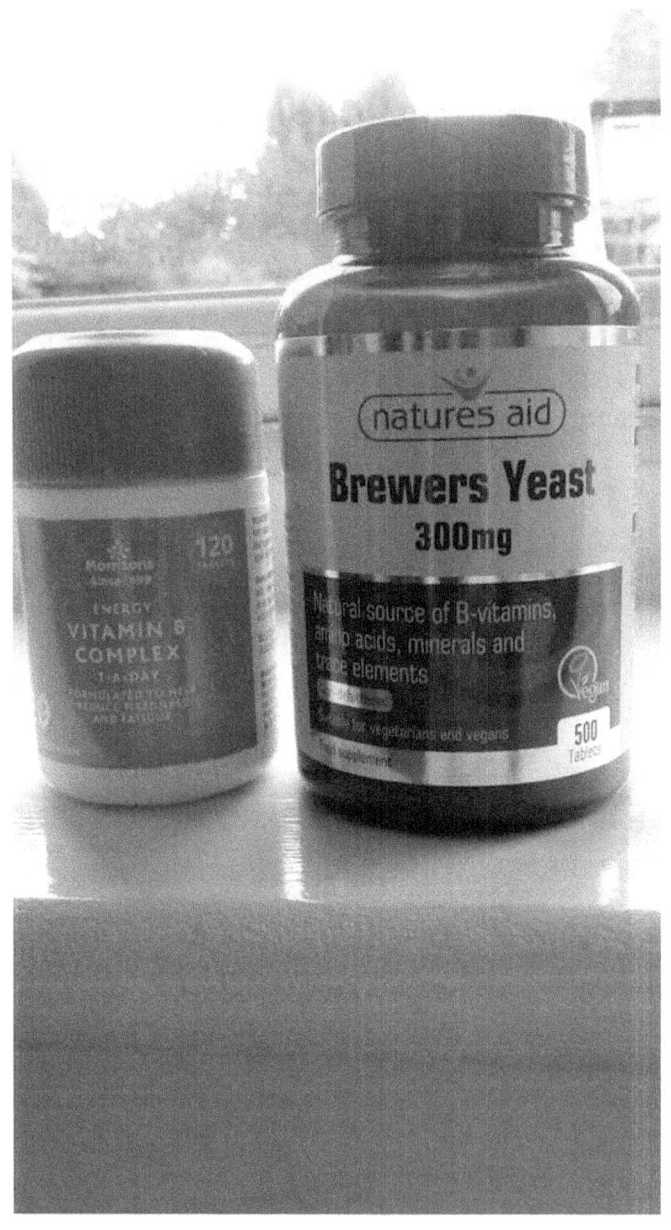

The benefits of Arginine

Arginine is an essential amino acid which means that it must be obtained from the diet as it cannot be made by the body.

In the body, arginine changes into nitric oxide. Nitric oxide is a neurotransmitter that helps blood vessels to relax. This also improves circulation and assists in lowering blood pressure. When the arteries are dilated and relaxed, blood flows better and this helps improve symptoms of clogged arteries, angina and coronary artery disease.

Arginine is found in good amounts in these dietary sources:

- Meat products
- Nuts and seeds
- Legumes

We should not forget the contribution of a group of poly unsaturated fatty acids – the omega 6's that are responsible for many of the inflammatory conditions that we live with nowadays.

It is to these that we will turn to now.

Pro and anti-inflammatory fats

The Good, the Bad and the Ugly about Fats and Oils

Ask most older people about saturated fats and they will be able to name a string of them at once. They were brought up on them. They formed part of the diet during the war and immediate post wars. They provided much needed calories and fat soluble vitamins that are often lacking in our diet.

Saturated fats are those fats which are solid at room temperature – butter, lard, dripping, meat and coconut oil are examples of saturated fat.

Saturated fats are another substance which have become demonised even though studies show that they raise HDL – the lipo-protein that is labelled 'good cholesterol'.

Saturated fat also changes the pattern of LDL, increasing the subgroup of LDL which transports much needed substances for cell growth and repair. Studies have shown that saturated fat is associated with less coronary atherosclerosis than it if it is replaced by other food groups.

When saturated fat is replaced with carbohydrate, for example, then the progression of atherosclerosis is greater. Further, when saturated fats are replaced with unsaturated fats, the progression of atherosclerosis also increases.

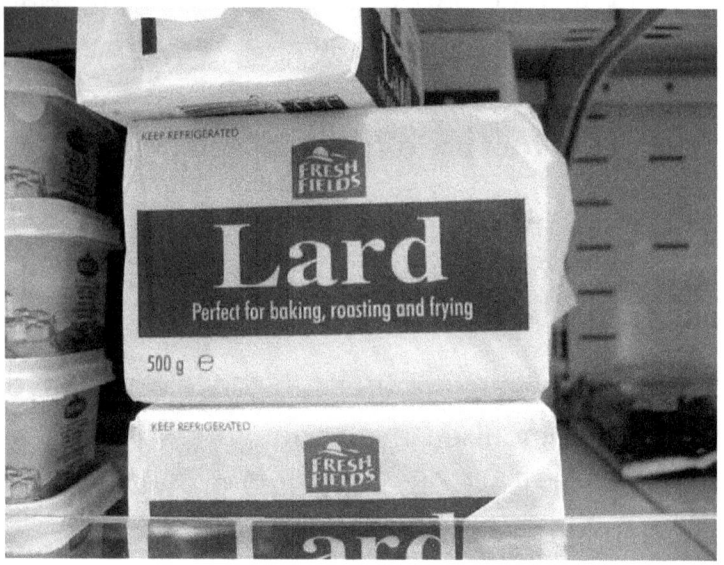

Lard could be considered a superfood. It is the second richest source of Vitamin D and is rich in cholesterol. It does not contain trans-fat – the real culprit behind heart disease and a major contributor to brain degeneration. It contains 60% monounsaturated fat which is associated with a decreased risk of heart disease. Monounsaturated fats also decrease inflammation. This is one of our prime tasks in the fight against neurodegeneration.

Saturated fat has many advantages over other fats for cooking. It is far more stable and so is less likely to be damaged when heated than, for example, oils such as olive oil or rape seed oil. This means it hardly generates free radicals that are implicated in the dementias.

Poly- unsaturated fatty acids.

A further group of fats - The poly unsaturated fats - are the omega 6's and the omega 3's - docosahexaenoic acid (DHA) and eicosapentoic acid (EPA). These are liquid at room temperature.

The polyunsaturated fatty acid found in omega six oils is called linoleic acid. It is derived from vegetable oils and it is a major player in fuelling inflammatory processes. Neurodegeneration and inflammation go hand in hand. Our diet is full of omega 6 without us realising it. These vegetable oils are added to just about every food on the market. It is hidden in biscuits and cakes, added to tinned soups etc.

it is now used for cooking fish and chips in when lard was once used.

Most of the population are not aware of how much ubiquitous pro-inflammatory oil they are ingesting. When it comes to saturated fat and omega 6, it cannot be repeated enough that it is the latter that creates inflammation.

Studies show that it is the balance between omega 6 and omega three which impacts far more on health than any concerns we may erroneously have about saturated fat. We should be eating far more omega 3 in our diet than we currently are and the amount of omega 6's should be limited significantly, if they have to be used.

Arichidonic acid is a polyunsaturated omega-6 fatty acid. It is found in the membranes of the body's cells and is particularly abundant in the brain, muscles and liver. It is a key inflammatory intermediate and can act as a vasodilator. This means it can widen blood vessels.

Arichidonic acid has many beneficial roles in the body. It will not cause inflammation unless tiny particles, called electrons, try and disrupt the stability of other electrons found in the fat that forms part of the cell membranes.

Arachidonic acid can be metabolised to both anti-inflammatory and proinflammatory eicanosoids. Eicanosoids are the end product of a series of metabolic processes. It is quite likely that if you suffer from joint pain, bronchoconstriction, microvascular permeability and lymphoedema that arachidonic acid has been converted to a pro-inflammatory compound.

There are numerous studies that show that arachidonic acid is implicated in Alzheimer's disease. Arachidonic acid activates enzymes called kinases. These kinases appear to increase tau phosphorylation levels. This just means that more phosphate is added to the tau protein that is characteristic of Alzheimer's disease.

Free arachidonic acid can be converted to substances that contribute to the occurrence and progression of neuroinflammation.[22]

Studies have shown that arachidonic acid is involved in bringing about the beta amyloid plaques in mouse models.

Essential fatty acids (EFA's) are vital for the health of the brain and regulate many of the processes that have been pathologically altered in Alzheimer's disease. These processes resulted in learning, memory and behavioural impairments in the mouse models.

While some nutrients can be made within the body, EFA's cannot. They have to be taken in through diet on a daily basis.

---

[22] https://www.jneurology.com/articles/arachidonic-acid-in-alzheimers-disease.html

Omega 3 fatty acids contain alpha linoleic acid which is found in walnuts and flaxseeds. It is an essential fatty acid. It is anti-inflammatory and good for reducing inflammation in arteries.

Two long chain omega three fatty acids that you should become familiar with are

- Eicosapentenoic acid (EPA) and
- Docosahexaenoic acid (DHA)

 As EPA and DHA can compete with arachidonic acid for the synthesis of eicosanoids then it is to our advantage that we take in more of these than arachidonic acid as they tip the balance towards less inflammatory activity.

There should be about six times the amount of omega 3's ingested to the omega 6's. The reality is that it is the other way around. We are eating far too many vegetable oils containing the pro-inflammatory omega 6 fatty acids. In other words, we are providing the fuel for a state of chronic inflammation including that involved in neurodegeneration.

The Victorians suffered very little heart disease in spite of their high saturated fat diet which was full of lard, dripping, eggs and butter. In fact, heart disease wasn't considered important enough to study at medical school in those times, since there was so little of it. Dementia is also a new disease on the block. We shall look at the reasons and evidence for this later.

Eventually these important saturated fats were replaced with the 'healthier' substitutes of.

- Omega 6 vegetable oils
- margarine

Crisco was one of the first new fats to be introduced to the unsuspecting public. It was promoted as making flakier pastry. It was full of trans fats. Trans fats are toxic to the human body.

Other important fats vital for brain and eye health are eggs.

Eggs were demonised as being full of 'bad' cholesterol. People were frightened to eat one of the most nutritionally and complete foods to be found.

The 'Go to work on an egg' was replaced by messages that eggs contained salmonella and should be avoided.

The junior minister – Edwina Currie – eventually had to resign from her post after the British Egg Industry Council called her remarks 'factually incorrect and highly irresponsible' saying that the risk of being infected with salmonella was less than 200 million to one.

Since saturated fats were replaced with 'healthier' substitutes, heart disease and neurodegenerative disease have increased markedly. Further, the introduction of cholesterol lowering drugs – which occurred more or less at the same time as these dietary changes - provide cogent explanations for the increase in chronic diseases.

Dr Weil M.D. in his book Healthy Aging observed that during the plenary presentations of the 11th Anti-Aging Conference and Exposition that it was mooted that chronic inflammation was a common root of neuro-degenerative disorders including Alzheimer disease, Parkinson's disease and Amyotrophic Sclerosis.

It was emphasised that dietary modifications were a treatment strategy – a view point which I also hold. However, it is unlikely to be promoted as a treatment strategy. It does not hold any profit for the pharmaceutical companies.

Monounsaturated fats help promote a healthy blood flow to the brain. They help to produce and release acetylcholine which is essential for learning and memory; the loss of acetylcholine will result in memory problems often associated with Alzheimer's disease.

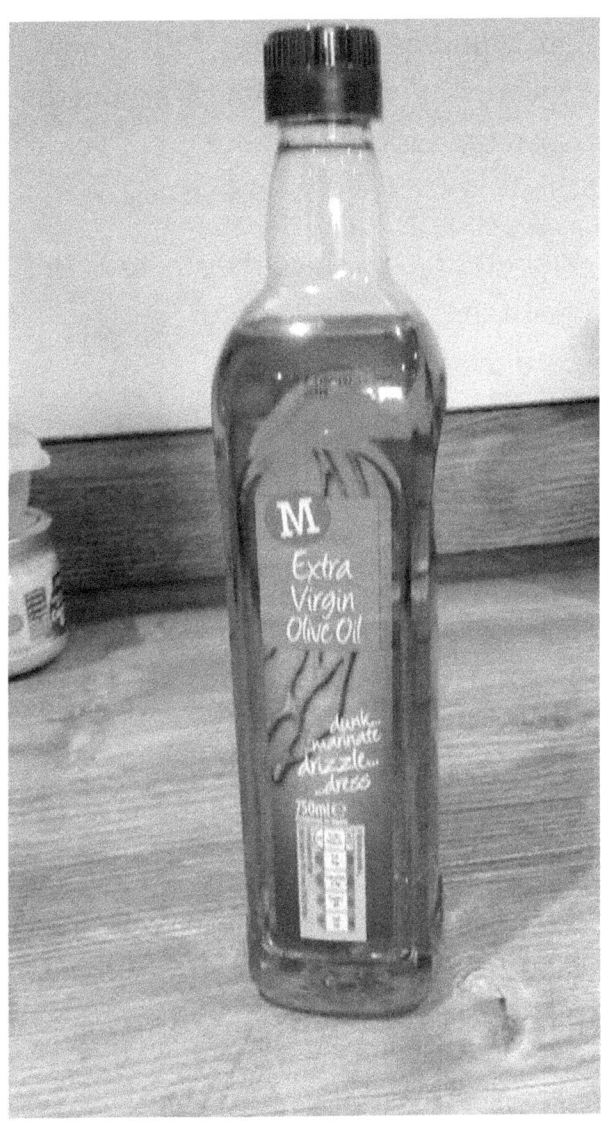

Olive oil reduces inflammation in arteries

There are a number of studies[23] that show that statins favour the metabolism of production of omega six fatty acids. The knock on effect of this is that this raises the risk of diseases like:

- diabetes type 2 since they increase insulin resistance
- cardiovascular disease
- brain disorders

By now you should have come to the realisation that cholesterol is regulated by the liver and does not need external assistance to lower it to levels which place it in a deficient state.

Cholesterol rises and falls in splendid rhythmicity responding to numerous states in the body that we will be entirely unaware of most of the time.

I know of no one who thinks to themselves, 'I need to make more hormones to cope with this stressful situation so my cholesterol levels will rise to cope with this situation.'

---

[23] https://www.ncbi.nlm.nih.gov/pmc/articles/PMC3571733/

I would prefer always that people ate sensibly to that excess cholesterol is swept away in the gut – something that oats and lentils and fibre do so well. This is the natural way that the body copes in addition to making sure that the liver is healthy and not functionally impaired through too much sugar and alcohol.

Although some saturated fat is good, we seem to have lost the concept of average amounts in a daily diet. 20g of saturated fat is about right for an adult. This equates to four teaspoons full.

However, those on a ketone diet where fat and protein are allowed do not appear to suffer problems if their saturated fat intake is greater than this.

Indeed, those on a ketogenic diet (similar to the Atkins diet) find that this reduces obesity, hypertension and lowers cholesterol levels.

Of course, not everyone can cope with a ketogenic diet and need slightly more carbohydrate than is recommended.

I make luxury oat breads. They are versatile, contain lots of trace elements like magnesium and potassium, soluble fibre, protein and do not contain added fat or sugar. They fill the hunger gaps very well.

I have given this recipe to a number of diabetics who don't want to give up the texture of bread but do not want to eat anything that may raise their blood sugar levels, either.

Not only has it stabilised their blood sugar levels but on every occasion their blood pressure had dropped to normal levels.

I suspect that this phenomenon is helped by the good quantities of potassium and magnesium in the mixture and the additional spice (I use cinnamon) which aids in lowering blood pressure too.

Here is one such recipe:

Banana Oat Bread

This is not a sweet cake. It is a luxury bread.
You can spread it with butter or jam or eat it by
itself. It is perfect for taking on long walks.

4 ripe bananas

1-2tsp of bicarbonate of soda

 3 - 4 eggs

Teaspoon of spice of your choice

Rolled oats about 400g

Milk or yogurt to mix

Method

Put the first 4 ingredients in a bowl and beat until it is battered (works better if you think of someone you don't like as you are doing it)

Add the oats and enough milk or yogurt to make a stiff mix. You can add extra oats or milk as needed.

Turn into a lined loaf tin and bake for 35 minutes at 180C until a knife inserted comes out clean. It may take longer

Variations

- Sometimes I chop up four windfall apples and substitute for the banana. I add extra spice   a handful of sultanas and sometimes ginger.
- You can add broken up chocolate to the basic banana mix
- Add chopped canned pineapple and desiccated coconut

- Half a tin of chopped tomatoes, some chopped olives and basil with grated cheese on the top before baking
- You can fold in mashed carrot instead of the banana with some walnuts and spread with cream cheese.

In fact, this is such a versatile recipe that it is limited only by your imagination.

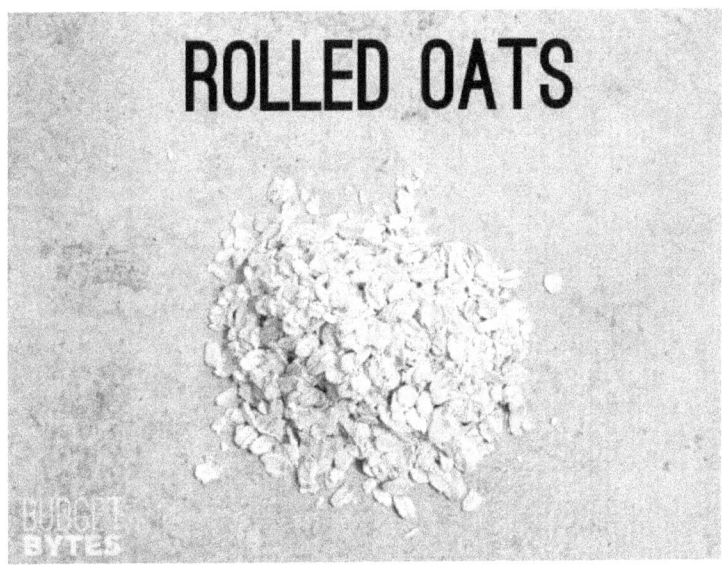

Rolled oats combine with other ingredients very well to make the perfect low fat, low GI bread

This is preferable to taking medications that not only reduce cholesterol but have a negative impact on other metabolic pathways at the same time.

Wrapping it all up

When we investigate the health of people who eat high fat/high cholesterol diets, we find that they tend to be healthy and do not easily suffer from infection. The Victorians enjoyed lavish helpings of cream, butter and cheese and yet were considered some of the healthiest people there were once infant mortality was taken out of the equation.

 For a long time, we have wondered at the 'French paradox' and what is behind it.

The French paradox is the observation that low coronary heart disease and low death rates occur despite a high intake of dietary cholesterol and saturated fat in the French diet. The mean energy supplied by fat is about 38% yet the incidence of obesity and coronary heart disease is extremely low.

The Atkins diet – in which you could eat as much fat as you liked – was effective in not only reducing weight but also reducing the risk of coronary heart disease. People did lose weight by eating a diet high in fat and did not suffer any associated high blood pressure or symptoms of cardiovascular disease. Neither fat nor cholesterol are responsible for the diseases that plague our society; the culprit is sugar.

Sugar contributes to inflammation in the artery walls. Every blood sugar spike, however, temporary, initiates sub clinical inflammation.

Sugar and processed carbohydrates raise triglycerides. Triglycerides are an independent risk factor for heart disease. When sugar attaches itself to proteins, it makes toxic molecules called advanced glycation end products also known as AGE's. This is a good acronym for they do speed the aging process.

Which fats are the healthy fats? Surprisingly, they are not the allegedly 'healthy' vegetable oils. The poly unsaturated fatty acid omega 6's also cause inflammation and should be avoided at all costs. These omega 6's are found in oils such as Canola and sunflower oil. They are used in many of the products that we buy in the supermarkets nowadays such as biscuits, flapjacks and similar baked products. Omega 6 fatty acids are also added to tinned soups and ready meals. Most ready prepared foods will have omega 6 oils added to them. It is good practice to get into the habit of reading the ingredients list on all processed foods in order to raise awareness of the ubiquitous nature of omega 6 fatty acids.

The stable fats are the saturated fats such as lard, dripping and butter. They generate very few free radicals and, as a consequence, are limited in their ability to cause inflammation.

 These are the fats that the French eat in fairly large amounts and the ones that the Victorians ate without restraint.

These fats contain vitamin D, support the immune system, allow absorption of vital fat soluble vitamins such as vitamin K and do not raise insulin levels. As such, saturated fats cannot cause weight gain as insulin is required to enable fat storage.

The risk of heart disease is not addressed through the use of statins or lowering cholesterol or saturated fat. It is addressed by including the nutrients that the body requires to keep arteries clean and dilated and free from inflammation. It does not take much effort to do this. Taking supplementary vitamin K2 is no more difficult than taking a statin. The former has positive benefits and the latter is fraught with problems.

Cholesterol does not generally need to be lowered through medical intervention unless you have a genetic disorder such as hypercholesterolemia.

Cholesterol levels will naturally fluctuate as they respond to the demands the body places on it.

The French paradox shows us that a diet that contains more than a third of saturated fat is a healthy one that will have a far reaching and positive impact on every aspect of our lives.

The rejection of statins as a medication that promotes health is long overdue. If statins did not impact other vital metabolic pathways, then

I would find them more acceptable in those who had a genuine genetic propensity to hypercholesterolemia.

Incident familial hypercholesterolemia is estimated at about one in three hundred. Some groups such as Finns, Ashkenazi Jews and Lebanese Christians appear to have a genetic propensity for this condition. In this case the incidence may rise as high as one in a hundred.

Should anyone still be in doubt about how diet impacts cholesterol and cardiovascular health then I have added details of a number of other studies below.

They will give you food for thought.

More Research

The Inuit have a diet that consists of 80% fat. However, they have healthy blood vessels.

[24]Another study examined the diets of Indians living in the north and south of India.

The Indians from the north ate lots of meat and ghee and had high cholesterol levels.

The Southern Indians ate a predominantly vegetarian diet with vegetable oil and margarine. They had lower cholesterol levels. These Indians had a 15 times greater incidence of heart disease than the meat/ghee eaters.

---

[24] American Journal of Clinical Nutrition, Rates of cardiovascular disease in N and S India 1967 20:462-475

List of soluble fibres

Oats

Peas

Beans

Carrots

Sweet potatoes

Barley

Psyllium husk

Prunes and figs

Citrus fruit

Mushroom

Avocado

Foods naturally high in dietary cholesterol

Kidneys and other organ meats such as liver

Eggs – one of the most nutritionally sound food that there are

Prawns

These foods do NOT impact blood cholesterol. Sugary foods, however, do.

The impact of fruit sugar in raising Very Low Density Lipoprotein should not be underestimated.

Useful Links

https://quintessentiallylynne.weebly.com/nutritional-medicine.html

https://www.amazon.co.uk/-/e/B07BPQZ5CD

https://authorcentral.amazon.com/gp/profile

Other Books that you may be interested in:

- **The Alzheimer's and Vascular Dementia Disease Diet**

https://www.amazon.com/dp/1082402850

- **Healing Shingles and Neuropathic Pain**

https://www.amazon.com/dp/1799040623

- **The MND Diet**

https://www.amazon.com/dp/B07K2FPX91

The Metabolic Syndrome Diet by Lynne D M Noble

Beat Hypertension Easily Using Nutrition by Lynne D M Noble

All available worldwide in either kindle or paperback form on Amazon

A percentage of the sale of these books is allocated for charitable purposes. One of the charity's that have benefitted from the sale of these books is

The Exodus Project

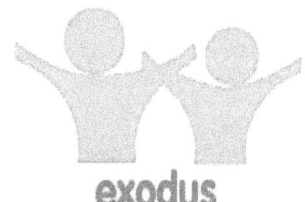

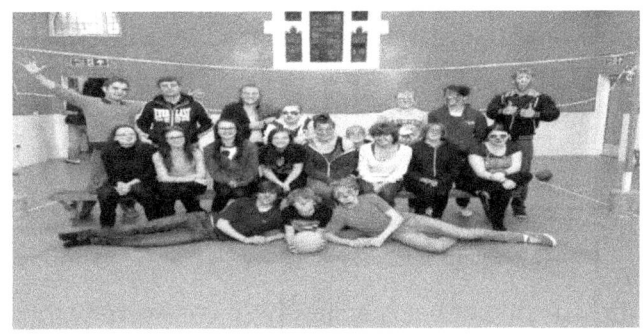

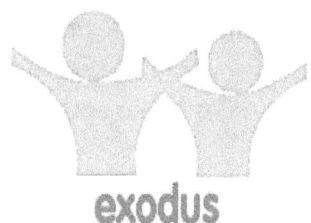

Exodus has been impacting the lives of children and young people in less advantaged communities for 20 years. Through a unique model of working, we build trusting relationships that create firm foundations for growing aspirations and regenerating communities. We target the most disadvantaged communities, trying to get kids to make the right choices for their lives.

We have learned that none of this will be achieved without long term commitment to the children and their families in these communities. Superficial remedies to deep rooted problems will only have short term impact. We are regarded as friends and not workers in the areas where we work. Our work is long established and our reputation for consistency and commitment is unquestioned. So what do we do?

We run mid-week activity clubs in the heart of the less advantaged communities of Barnsley. We bus in equipment and volunteers, to join local people in delivering exciting and fast moving activity programmes for the local kids. The programmes are great fun, as well as educational. We do dance, drama, craft, music, sports and games to entertain and energise. We also talk to the kids about the issues going on in their communities. So, if the local allotments have been broken into, or kids have been playing football on the bowling green again, we can discuss anti-social behaviour and attitudes with examples that the local young people identify with.

As well as activity clubs and home visits we take the kids away on activity weekends. We have our own activity centre, known as Jenny's Field, which we use for these weekend retreats. Jenny's Field is a home from home and a place of refuge and encouragement for so many children and young people.

The final aspect of our work might generally be termed "community partnerships". We don't want to work in isolation and we partner with parents and carers, local residents' associations, the police, housing authorities, schools and others to ensure a coordinated approach to issues on the estates.

Perhaps the most rewarding aspect of our work is the development of junior volunteers. Many of the young people who come through the activity clubs structure continue their involvement with us as leaders in the clubs where they were once members. Over the years we have nurtured hundreds of young people, sustaining relationships with them throughout their turbulent teenage years. Joe says it best:

"I very quickly fell into the family of Exodus. At such a young age nothing in my life was certain, but I knew that I belonged here. I've gone from a gobby little kid, who used to spend hours in a porch, to a not much bigger adult with a remarkable story to tell, of how God has guided and supported me and lead me down the right path, when it would have been so easy to stray."

Facebook: TheExodusProjectBarnsley

www. exodusproject.org.uk